BREAST CANCER DIET FOR BEGINNERS

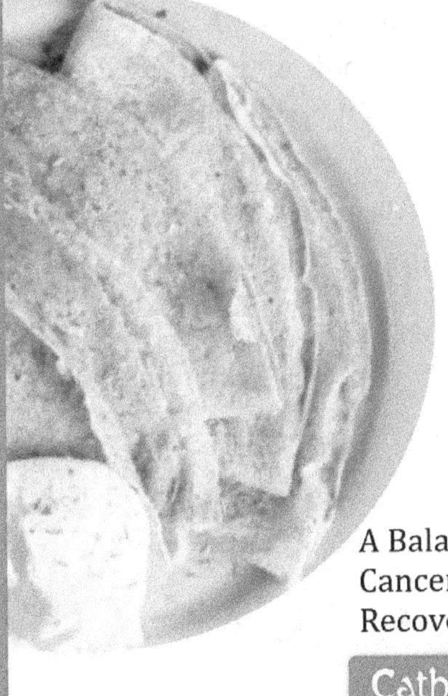

BONUS

14 DAY MEAL PLAN PLUS 20 DAY MEAL PLANNER INCLUDED

A Balanced Diet For Breast Cancer Prevention And Recovery

Cathryn D. Dutton

ABSTRACT

The "Breast Cancer Diet Cookbook for Beginners" offers a comprehensive collection of nourishing recipes tailored to support individuals navigating the challenges of breast cancer. This cookbook combines accessible culinary guidance with evidence-based nutritional insights, making it an essential resource for those seeking to enhance their well-being during their cancer journey. From wholesome meal ideas to dietary tips, the cookbook empowers beginners to make informed food choices that contribute to their overall health and vitality. With a focus on balance and flavor, this cookbook encourages a positive relationship with food while promoting nutrition that aligns with the needs of breast cancer patients.

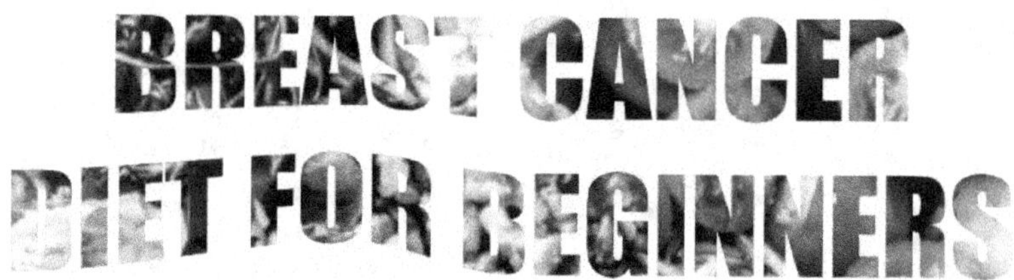

TABLE OF CONTENTS

BREAST CANCER DIET FOR BEGINNERS

INTRODUCTION

Emily had always been an avid reader, but after learning that her mother had breast cancer, she began to read for a different reason. Emily started researching diet and cancer because she was determined to do anything she could to support her mother. She searched online databases and libraries for research before discovering a book titled "Breast Cancer Diet for Beginners."

Emily read the book cover to cover, taking in every piece of wisdom it had. She discovered the value of eating a well-balanced diet that is high in antioxidants and low in processed foods. She found meals that were both scrumptious and nutritious. Emily improved her family's meals using the knowledge she had just learned.

Her mother's health became better as the months went by. Her physicians expressed their admiration for the improvement and gave Emily credit for her mother's improved diet. In addition to helping her mother, Emily's transition from voracious reader to caregiver gave her a new mission in life: raising awareness of the critical importance of nutrition in cancer treatment.

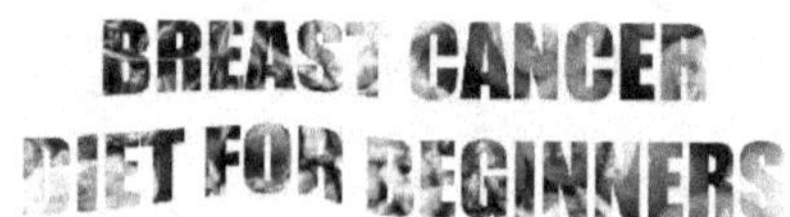

I'd be happy to help! While there's no single food that can prevent or control cancer, a balanced and healthy diet can contribute to overall well-being. Here are 10 breakfast recipe ideas that include cancer-fighting ingredients:

1. Berry Smoothie Bowl

Ingredients:

- 1 cup of mixed berries, including raspberries, blueberries, and strawberries
- one ripe banana
- Greek yogurt, half a cup
- 1/4 cup milk, either dairy or vegan
- rolled oats, two teaspoons
- 1 tablespoon of maple syrup or honey
- Choose your own toppings (fruit slices, nuts, seeds, granola, or coconut flakes).

Preparation

1. Slice the banana and wash the mixed berries.
2. Blend the mixed berries, banana, milk, rolled oats, honey, or maple syrup in a food processor.
3. Blend till creamy and smooth. Add a bit more milk if the mixture is too thick.
4. Mixture should be poured into a bowl.

5. Put the toppings you choose on top of the smoothie. Here, you can be creative and incorporate granola, sliced fruit, nuts, seeds, and coconut flakes.

Enjoy your delectable Berry Smoothie Bowl right away.

2.Oatmeal with Flaxseeds

Ingredients

- rolled oats, 1 cup
- 2 cups of water or milk, either dairy or vegan
- flaxseeds, two tablespoons
- Sliced bananas, berries, honey, almonds, and cinnamon are optional toppings.

Preparation

1. Bring the milk or water to a medium boil in a saucepan.

2. Turn the heat down to medium-low after stirring in the rolled oats. Allow it to simmer for about 5 minutes, stirring regularly, or until the oats are cooked to the desired consistency.

3. While the oats are cooking, you may toast the flaxseeds for about two to three minutes, stirring often, in a dry skillet over medium heat. They taste more nutty as a result.

4. When the oats are done cooking, turn off the heat and add the flaxseeds that have been toasted.

5. Give the oatmeal a few minutes to thicken.

6. Serve the oats in bowls and top with your favorite ingredients, such as sliced bananas, berries, nuts, honey, or cinnamon.

Enjoy your flaxseed-infused, nutrient-rich oatmeal!

3. Avocado Toast

Ingredients

- 1 mature avocado
- 2 slices of whole grain (or other type of) bread
- pepper and salt as desired
- Red pepper flakes, sliced tomatoes, a poached egg, feta cheese, and other optional toppings.

Preparation

1. Remove the avocado's pit, cut it in half, and scoop the flesh into a bowl.

2. Use a fork to mash the avocado until it is as creamy as you like. You may either make it smooth or leave it slightly lumpy.

3. The bread pieces should be crisp and golden brown after toasting.

4. Over the toasted bread slices, evenly distribute the mashed avocado.

5. On top of the avocado, season with salt and pepper to taste.

6. Add any extra toppings you'd want, if you'd like. Sliced tomatoes, red pepper flakes for heat, a poached egg for extra protein, or feta cheese crumbles for taste are a few examples.

7. The avocado toast should be served right away.

4. Greek Yogurt Parfait

Ingredients

- Greek yogurt, one cup
- 14 cup of granola
- 1 cup of mixed berries, including raspberries, blueberries, and strawberries
- 2 teaspoons of maple syrup or honey
- (Optional) 1/4 teaspoon vanilla extract

1. Wash and slice the strawberries if necessary to prepare the berries. Other berries, such as blueberries and raspberries, can be added. Put them apart.

2. The yogurt should be thoroughly blended with the honey, maple syrup, and vanilla extract (if using) in a bowl. The yogurt will become sweeter and more flavorful as a result.

3. The Greek yogurt mixture should be layered, beginning at the bottom of the serving glass or dish.

4. Add Granola: Cover the yogurt with a layer of granola. This will give the food more crunch and nutty flavor.

5. Add Berries: Top the granola with a layer of mixed berries. A variety of berries can be used to provide color and freshness.

6. Repeat Layers: Continue adding layers until all the ingredients have been utilized, ending with a final layer of berries on top.

7. It's time to enjoy your Greek yogurt parfait! You may either serve it right away or, if you prefer it slightly cooled, put it in the refrigerator for a short period.

8. Optional Variations: To add extra texture and taste to your parfait, you can add other ingredients like chopped almonds, chia seeds, or shredded coconut in between the layers.

5. Chia Seed Pudding

Ingredients

1. Chia seeds, 1/4 cup
2. 1 cup milk, either dairy or vegan
3. 1-2 teaspoons of sweetener (such as honey, agave, maple syrup, etc.)
4. 0.5 teaspoons of optional vanilla extract
5. Toppings for fresh fruit, nuts, or granola are optional.

Preparation Method

1. Chia seeds and milk should be mixed in a bowl. Stir thoroughly to make sure the chia seeds are dispersed uniformly and aren't clumped together.

2. Add vanilla extract and sweetener to the mixture. To combine everything, stir it once more.

3. Refrigerate the bowl for at least 4 hours or overnight. Cover it with plastic wrap or a lid. This enables the chia seeds to absorb the liquid and take on the consistency of pudding.

4. Give the mixture a brisk swirl once it has hardened to remove any clumps and ensure a smooth texture.

5. Chia seed pudding should be served in bowls or glasses. For more taste and texture, sprinkle some fresh fruit, nuts, or granola on top.

Enjoy the chia seed pudding you cooked at home!

6. Spinach and Mushroom Egg Scramble

Ingredients

- 2 cups freshly cleaned and sliced spinach
- 1 cup sliced mushrooms
- 4 eggs
- 14 cup of milk
- pepper and salt as desired
- 1 tablespoon of cooking oil or butter
- Grated cheese (feta, mozzarella, or cheddar) is optional.

Preparation Method

1. Melt the butter or add cooking oil to a skillet that has been preheated to medium heat.
2. Sliced mushrooms should be added to the skillet and cooked for two to three minutes, or until they begin to brown and release moisture.

3. To the skillet, add the chopped spinach, and cook for an additional two minutes, or until the spinach wilts.

4. Whisk the eggs, milk, salt, and pepper in a bowl.

5. Over the cooked spinach and mushrooms in the skillet, pour the egg mixture.

6. With a spatula, gently mix and scramble the eggs, moving them about the skillet as they cook.

7. When the eggs are totally cooked but still slightly creamy, keep heating and stirring. It ought to take three to four minutes.

8. You can sprinkle grated cheese over the scrambled eggs and let it melt if you're using it.

9. Remove the skillet from the heat once the eggs are done to your preference.

10. Serve the hot spinach and mushroom egg scramble with optional extra fresh herbs or cheese on top as a garnish.

11. Take pleasure in your savory and nourishing Spinach and Mushroom Egg Scramble!

7. Salmon Breakfast Wrap

Ingredients

- 1 significant whole-wheat tortilla
- Salmon, smoked or cooked, 4 ounces
- two huge eggs
- sliced red onion, diced tomato, diced cucumber, and 1/4 cup
- a serving of cream cheese, two
- 1 tablespoon finely sliced fresh dill
- pepper and salt as desired
- cooking spray or oil for frying

Preparation Method

1. Salt and pepper the eggs in a bowl after whisking them.

2. Add a tiny amount of frying oil or non-stick cooking spray to a non-stick skillet that is already heated over medium heat.

3. When the eggs are scrambled to the proper consistency, pour the whisked eggs into the skillet. Get rid of the heat.

4. On a spotless surface, spread out the whole wheat tortilla.

5. A border of about an inch should be left around the tortilla's borders as you spread the cream cheese evenly over it.

6. Place a line of scrambled eggs down the middle of the tortilla.

7. Over the eggs, place the cooked or smoked salmon.

8. Over the salmon, scatter the diced red onion, tomato, and cucumber.

9. If using, scatter fresh dill that has been chopped over the vegetables.

10. The sides of the tortilla should be folded in before being securely rolled up to enclose the filling.

11. You can choose to microwave the wrap for 20 to 30 seconds

12. to slightly melt the cream cheese and rewarm the contents.

13. Serve the salmon breakfast wrap right away, whole or split in half for convenience.

8. Turmeric Scrambled Tofu

Ingredients

- 1 block (14 oz) of crumbled, drained firm tofu
- 1 teaspoon of turmeric, ground

- 1/8 teaspoon cumin powder
- 1/8 teaspoon coriander powder
- An optional 1/4 teaspoon of black salt (kala namak), for an eggy flavor
- To taste, add salt and pepper.
- 1 tablespoon oil (either neutral oil or olive oil)
- 1/2 onion, chopped finely
- finely sliced half a bell pepper
- 2 minced garlic cloves
- Two tablespoons of nutritional yeast
- chopped fresh cilantro or parsley (for garnish)

Preparation Method

1. To start, drain the tofu. To assist press out extra moisture, set the tofu block on a plate, cover with a paper towel, place another plate on top, and then weight it down with a can or other large object. Allow it to sit for 15 to 20 minutes.

2. Prepare the seasoning while the tofu is draining. Combine the ground turmeric, cumin, coriander, black salt (if using), salt, and pepper in a small bowl. Place aside.

3. Once the tofu has been thoroughly drained, break it up with your hands.

4. A big skillet with medium heat is used to heat the oil. Add the diced bell pepper and onion. They should soften after 3–4 minutes of sautéing.

5. Tofu crumbles and minced garlic are added to the skillet. With the vegetables in the pan, stir to mix.

6. The tofu and vegetables should be covered with the spice mixture. To distribute the spices evenly, thoroughly stir. Cook the tofu for a further 5-7 minutes, stirring periodically, or until it is thoroughly cooked and beginning to become brown.

7. If using, add nutritional yeast to the dish and whisk to incorporate.

8. If necessary, taste and adjust the seasoning.

9. Remove from heat once everything is cooked and seasoned to your preferences.

10. Add chopped parsley or cilantro as a garnish.

11. As a savory supper or a protein-rich breakfast, serve the warm turmeric scrambled tofu.

12. Enjoy your flavorful and nutritious Turmeric Scrambled Tofu!

9.Whole-Grain Pancakes

Ingredients

- whole wheat flour, 1 cup
- a spoonful of optional sugar
- one tablespoon of baking powder
- A half-teaspoon of baking soda
- 1 cup buttermilk (or other milk of your choice) and 1/4 teaspoon salt
- 1 egg
- 2 tablespoons of melted oil or butter
- 1 teaspoon optional vanilla extract

Preparation

1. Mix the whole wheat flour, salt, baking soda, baking powder, and sugar (if using) in a mixing dish.

2. Beat the egg in a different basin, and then stir in the buttermilk, melted butter, and vanilla extract (if using). Mix thoroughly.

3. After adding the liquid ingredients, combine the dry ingredients by gently combining them. Even a few bumps are OK.

4. Give the batter five to ten minutes to rest. This makes the pancakes fluffier by facilitating the whole wheat flour's absorption of the liquid.

5. A nonstick griddle or skillet should be heated to medium. If necessary, you might give it a small coating of butter or oil.

6. For each pancake, pour 1/4 cup of batter into the griddle.

7. Cook for two to three minutes, or until the pancake surface begins to bubble and the edges start to look set.

8. The pancakes should cook for an additional 1-2 minutes, or until golden brown, after being carefully flipped.

9. Pancakes should be taken off of the skillet and kept warm.

10. Use the leftover batter to complete the process, adding more butter or oil to the skillet as necessary.

With your preferred toppings, such as maple syrup, fruit, yogurt, or nuts, serve the whole-grain pancakes.

10.Fruit Salad with Nuts

Ingredients

- a variety of fresh fruits (including bananas, strawberries, blueberries, kiwis, grapes, and oranges)
- nuts of your preference (such as pecans, walnuts, or almonds)
- (Optional, for drizzling) Honey or maple syrup

- Fresh mint leaves can be used as a garnish.

Preparation Method

1. As necessary, wash and peel the fruits. Put them in a mixing dish after cutting them into bite-sized pieces.

2. A few nuts should be added to the bowl. Depending on your preference, you can either chop them roughly or leave them whole.

3. Make sure the fruits and nuts are distributed evenly by giving them a gentle toss.

4. Pour honey or maple syrup over the salad, as desired, to give it more sweetness. You can change the quantity to suit your preferences.

5. Remix the salad to evenly distribute the sweetener over the fruits and nuts.

6. If using, rip some fresh mint leaves into pieces and sprinkle them on top for a splash of flavor and color.

7. The fruit salad can be served right away or chilled in the fridge before serving.

8. To promote your general health, keep in mind the importance of eating a varied diet that includes lots of fruits, vegetables, whole grains, lean proteins, and

healthy fats. A healthcare expert should always be consulted for individualized dietary guidance.

Certainly! Here are 10 lunch recipe ideas that incorporate cancer-fighting ingredients:

1.Grilled Vegetable Salad.

here's a basic recipe for a Grilled Vegetable Salad:

Ingredients

- a variety of veggies (including cherry tomatoes, red onions, bell peppers, zucchini, and eggplant)
- Almond oil
- Pepper and salt
- vinegar of balsam
- Fresh herbs (such thyme, basil, or parsley)
- mixed greens (such as arugula, spinach, or lettuce)
- Feta cheese crumbles, roasted pine nuts, or sliced almonds are optional.

Preparation

1. A grill or grill pan should be preheated to high heat.

2. For even grilling, wash and slice the vegetables into uniform pieces.

3. Sliced veggies should be equally coated with olive oil, salt, and pepper in a bowl.

4. Vegetables should be grilled until they have attractive grill marks and are tender, flipping them occasionally. Depending on the variety and thickness of the vegetable, this could take 5 to 10 minutes.

5. After being grilled, take the vegetables off the heat and give

6. them a moment to cool.

7. Mix the grilled veggies and mixed greens in a big bowl.

8. Add a little more olive oil and balsamic vinegar. Toss everything together and evenly coat it.

9. For more taste, top the salad with fresh herbs.

10. To add more texture and flavor to the salad, you can sprinkle some crumbled feta cheese, toasted pine nuts, or sliced almonds on top.

11. Serve the grilled vegetable salad as a side dish or, to make it a full dinner, add some protein (grilled chicken, shrimp, or tofu).

2. Mediterranean Chickpea Bowl

Ingredients

For the chickpeas:

- 2 cans (15 oz each) of rinsed and drained chickpeas
- Olive oil, two tablespoons
- 1 teaspoon of cumin, ground
- 1 paprika teaspoon
- pepper and salt as desired

For the bowl

- Cooked quinoa or brown rice, 2 cups
- 1 cup halved cherry tomatoes, 1 cup diced cucumber, 1 cup thinly sliced red onion, and 1/2 cup pitted and sliced Kalamata olives
- 1/2 cup feta cheese crumbles
- chopped fresh parsley for a garnish

For the dressing

- Extra virgin olive oil, 1/4 cup
- Lemon juice, two tablespoons
- 1 minced garlic clove
- Oregano, dry, 1 teaspoon
- pepper and salt as desired

Preheat the oven to 400°F (200°C).

1. The drained chickpeas, olive oil, cumin, paprika, salt, and pepper should all be combined in a mixing bowl. Stir until the spices are coated evenly on the chickpeas.

2. On a baking sheet, arrange the seasoned chickpeas in a single layer. Until the chickpeas are crispy and golden, roast in the preheated oven for 20 to 25 minutes, shaking the pan halfway through.

3. While the chickpeas are roasting, prepare the dressing. In a small bowl, whisk together the extra-virgin olive oil, lemon juice, minced garlic, dried oregano, salt, and pepper. Place aside.

4. Place cooked quinoa or brown rice, roasted chickpeas, cherry tomatoes, diced cucumber, sliced red onion, Kalamata olives, and crumbled feta cheese in each serving dish to make the Mediterranean chickpea bowls.

5. Dressing should be drizzled over the assembled bowls.

6. Add freshly cut parsley as a garnish.

Enjoy the Mediterranean chickpea bowls right now. !

3. Broccoli and Almond Stir-Fry

Ingredients

- 200 grams of broccoli florets
- Sliced almonds in a cup
- Vegetable oil, two tablespoons
- 2 minced garlic cloves
- 1 teaspoon of ginger, grated
- 2/fourths cup soy sauce
- 1 optional tablespoon of oyster sauce
- pepper and salt as desired
- (Optional) Red pepper flakes for heat
- garnishing with sesame seeds

Preparation

1. Broccoli florets should be blanched in boiling water for around two minutes before being immediately transferred to ice water to stop the cooking process. Drain, then set apart.
2. Heat the vegetable oil over medium-high heat in a big skillet or wok.
3. Sliced almonds should be added to the skillet and stir-fried until golden brown. Almonds should be removed and put aside.

4. Add the minced garlic and grated ginger to the same skillet. Stir-fry until aromatic for around 30 seconds.

5. Broccoli florets that have been blanched should be added to the skillet and stir-fried for an additional 2-3 minutes, or until tender-crisp.

6. The soy sauce and oyster sauce (if using) should be added to the area that was left empty after pushing the broccoli to the side of the skillet. Stirring while allowing the sauces to warm up briefly.

7. After thoroughly combining the sauces, toss in the broccoli. If preferred, add red pepper flakes, salt, and pepper to taste.

8. Give the mixture one last swirl before adding the roasted almonds back to the skillet.

9. Transfer to a serving dish after taking it off the heat.

10. Garnish with sesame seeds before serving.

4. Lentil and Spinach Soup

Ingredients

- 1 cup of drained and rinsed green or brown lentils
- 1 chopped onion, 2 minced garlic cloves, 2 diced carrots, 2 diced celery stalks, and 4 cups of vegetable or chicken broth
- 1 can (14 oz) shredded tomatoes
- 2 cups chopped fresh spinach leaves
- 1 teaspoon of cumin, ground
- 1 teaspoon of coriander, ground
- Half a teaspoon of turmeric
- To taste-tested salt and pepper Olive oil for sautéing

Preparation Method

1. Add a drizzle of olive oil to a big saucepan that's heating up over medium heat.

2. Sauté the minced garlic and finely diced onion till transparent and fragrant.

3. Cook the diced carrots and celery for a few more minutes, or until they begin to soften.

4. Add the salt, pepper, turmeric, ground cumin, and ground coriander. To toast the spices, cook for one more minute.

5. Lentils that have been rinsed, chicken or vegetable broth, and diced tomatoes with juices should all be added to the saucepan. The mixture should boil.

6. When the lentils are ready, turn the heat down to low, cover the pot, and simmer the soup for 20 to 25 minutes.

7. Stir the saucepan while adding the chopped spinach until it wilts.

8. If necessary, taste the soup and adjust the seasoning.

9. Serve the hot lentil and spinach soup with a dollop of yogurt or a drizzle of olive oil as an optional garnish.

The handmade lentil and spinach soup is delicious.
!

BREAST CANCER
DIET FOR BEGINNERS

5. Salmon and Quinoa Bowl

Ingredients

- 2 fillets of salmon
- quinoa, one cup
- 2 cups of chicken broth or water
- 1 cup of chopped mixed veggies, including broccoli, carrots, and bell peppers
- Olive oil, two tablespoons
- pepper and salt as desired
- serving slices of lemon
- Avocado slices, chopped herbs (such parsley or cilantro), and sesame seeds are optional garnishes.

Preparation

1. In order to get rid of any bitterness, rinse the quinoa in cold water.

2. The rinsed quinoa should be combined with water or chicken broth in a medium pot. Bring to a boil, then lower the heat to a simmer, cover the pan, and cook the quinoa for 15 to 20 minutes, or until it is cooked and the liquid has been absorbed. With a fork, fluff the quinoa and set it aside.

3. Set the oven's temperature to 400°F (200°C).

4. Salmon fillets should be put on a baking pan covered with parchment paper. Sprinkle with salt and pepper and drizzle with olive oil.

5. When the salmon flakes easily with a fork, bake the salmon in the preheated oven for 12 to 15 minutes.

6. A tablespoon of olive oil should be heated over medium heat in a skillet while the salmon is roasting. Add the chopped vegetables and cook them until they are soft but have retained some of their crispness. To taste, add salt and pepper to the food.

7. Divide the cooked quinoa among serving dishes to assemble the bowls. Add the baked salmon fillets and sautéed veggies on top.

8. Add optional toppings to the bowls, including avocado slices, minced herbs, and sesame seeds.

9. Lemon wedges should be placed on the side of the bowls for squeezing over the salmon.

10. Take pleasure in your satisfying and wholesome Salmon and Quinoa Bowl!

6. Kale and Walnut Salad

Ingredients

- 4 cups of washed, de-stemmed, and chopped kale leaves
- 1 cup, roughly chopped walnuts
- 1/2 cup raisins or cranberries that are dried
- Feta cheese crumbles, 1/4 cup (optional)
- 1/4 cup finely sliced red onion
- Olive oil, 1/4 cup
- Lemon juice, two tablespoons
- 1 tablespoon of maple syrup or honey
- pepper and salt as desired

Preparation

1. The chopped kale, walnuts, dried cranberries or raisins, feta cheese, and thinly sliced red onion should all be combined in a big bowl.

2. Olive oil, lemon juice, honey or maple syrup, salt, and pepper should all be thoroughly blended in a separate small basin.

3. Toss the ingredients together until the kale leaves are thoroughly covered in the dressing after adding the dressing to the kale combination.

4. To allow the flavors to mingle and the kale to slightly soften, let the salad sit for 10 to 15 minutes.

5. Prior to serving, give the salad one last toss. If necessary, you can change the seasoning.

6. Serve the kale and walnut salad as a side dish or turn it into a full meal by adding grilled chicken, tofu, or chickpeas.

7. Take pleasure in your wholesome and delicious Kale and Walnut Salad.

7. Tuna and White Bean Salad

Ingredients

- 1 can (15 ounces) of washed and drain white beans (cannellini or Great Northern).
- 1 can (5-6 ounces) of flaked and drained tuna
- 1/2 red onion, chopped finely
- Half a cup of cherry tomatoes
- 14 cup finely minced fresh parsley
- (Optional) 1/4 cup finely chopped fresh basil
- Olive oil, two tablespoons
- one teaspoon of lemon juice
- pepper and salt as desired

1. White beans, flaked tuna, chopped red onion, cherry tomatoes, chopped parsley, and basil (if used) should all be combined in a big bowl.

2. The dressing is made by combining the olive oil, lemon juice, salt, and pepper in a small bowl.

3. Over the bean and tuna mixture, drizzle the dressing. Make sure all of the ingredients are coated in the dressing by giving everything a little toss to incorporate.

4. If necessary, add additional salt, pepper, or lemon juice after tasting and adjusting the seasoning.

5. To allow the flavors to mingle, let the salad sit for 10 to 15 minutes.

6. The Tuna and White Bean Salad can be served as a main course or a side dish. It goes well on its own, with some crusty bread, or over a bed of greens.

7. Take pleasure in your savory and nourishing tuna and white bean salad.

8.Veggie Wrap with Hummus

Ingredients

- (Whole wheat or your preferred type of tortilla)
- (Homemade or store-bought) hummus
- a variety of vegetables, including red onion, carrots, bell peppers, lettuce, and cucumber
- optional extras (olives, feta cheese, avocado slices, etc.)
- pepper and salt as desired

Preparation Method

1. Wash and prep each vegetable. Cucumber, bell peppers, carrots, and red onion should all be thinly sliced. Lettuce leaves should be washed and torn.

2. On a spotless surface, spread out a tortilla wrap.

3. Leave a little border of space around the edges as you generously spread hummus across the tortilla's center.

4. On top of the hummus, arrange the cut vegetables and any additional ingredients.

5. To add taste, season with a pinch of salt and pepper.

6. The tortilla should be folded in at the sides before being tightly rolled up, beginning at the bottom, to create a wrap.

7. To keep the wrap together while eating, if desired, use foil or parchment paper.

8. For the additional wraps, follow the same procedure.

9. You can either serve the Veggie Wraps with Hummus right away or, if you prefer, you may wrap them in plastic wrap and chill them for a few hours before serving.

Enjoy your savory and nourishing hummus-filled veggie wrap!

9. Brown Rice Sushi Rolls

Ingredients

- 2 cups of brown rice, cooked
- Rice vinegar, two tablespoons
- 1 teaspoon salt and 2 tablespoons sugar
- Nori sheets of seaweed
- various fillings, including imitation crab, grilled shrimp, avocado, and cucumber
- For dipping, soy sauce
- Ginger pickles and wasabi are optional.

1. In a small bowl, mix the rice vinegar, sugar, and salt until the sugar and salt dissolve.

2. Brown rice that has been cooked and the substance added should be combined gradually. Give it time to reach room temperature.

3. On a spotless surface, spread a bamboo sushi rolling mat and cover it with plastic wrap. Lay a nori seaweed sheet on the plastic wrap with the shiny side facing up.

4. Spread a thin layer of the prepared brown rice evenly over

5. the nori, moistening your fingers with water to prevent sticking, leaving about an inch of the nori sheet exposed at the top.

6. Choose your fillings and distribute them horizontally down the middle of the nori sheet covered in rice.

7. Start rolling the nori sheet onto the bamboo mat from the bottom, applying light pressure to form a tight cylinder.

8. Once the nori sheet has been rolled, wet the exposed edge with a little water to seal the roll.

9. Cut the roll into bite-sized pieces with a sharp knife.

10. Apply the remaining materials and repeat the procedure.

11. Sushi made with brown rice should be served with soy
    sauce on the side. Additionally, you can provide wasabi
    and pickled ginger alongside them.

12. Take pleasure in your homemade brown rice sushi!

10. Black Bean and Sweet Potato Burrito

Ingredients

- two medium sweet potatoes, diced after being peeled
- 1 can (15 oz) washed and drained black beans
- 1 cup of brown rice, cooked
- 1 chopped tiny onion
- 2 minced garlic cloves
- 1/9 cup cumin
- one tablespoon of chili powder
- pepper and salt as desired
- 4 substantial whole-wheat tortillas
- 1 cup of grated cheese (your choice of cheddar, monterey
  jack, or both)
- Optional garnishes: chopped cilantro, sour cream, salsa,
  and guacamole

Preparation

Preheat your oven to 400°F (200°C).

1. On a baking pan, arrange the sweet potatoes in dice. Add a little oil, then season with salt and pepper. The sweet potatoes should be roasted in the preheated oven for 20 to 25 minutes, or until they are soft and the edges are just starting to get crispy.

2. A little oil should be heated in a skillet over medium heat. Cook the onion till transparent after adding it.
3. Cumin, chili powder, and minced garlic are added to the skillet. Cook until aromatic for approximately 1 minute.

4. Black beans should be added to the skillet. Stir and heat well for a few minutes. If you want a creamier texture, you can mash some of the beans with the back of a spoon.

5. Add the cooked brown rice and sweet potatoes after stirring. Everything should be combined and cooked for a few more minutes to get the desired temperature. To taste, add salt and pepper to the food.

6. To soften the whole wheat tortillas, warm them in a dry skillet or briefly zap them in the microwave.

7. Put a dollop of the sweet potato and black bean mixture in the middle of each tortilla before putting the burritos together. Add some cheese shredded on top and any additional toppings you choose.
8. To form a burrito, fold the tortilla's sides in and then roll it up from the bottom.

9. The burritos can either be served as is, or you can lightly crisp the tortilla and melt the cheese by frying it in a hot skillet for a few seconds on each side.

10. If preferred, top the burritos with extra ingredients such salsa, guacamole, sour cream, and chopped cilantro.

Enjoy your Black Bean and Sweet Potato Burritos!

To maintain a balanced and nutrient-dense diet, always put an emphasis on including a range of vegetables, whole grains, lean meats, and healthy fats in your meals. A healthcare practitioner you consult with can offer you individualized advice based on your particular health requirements.

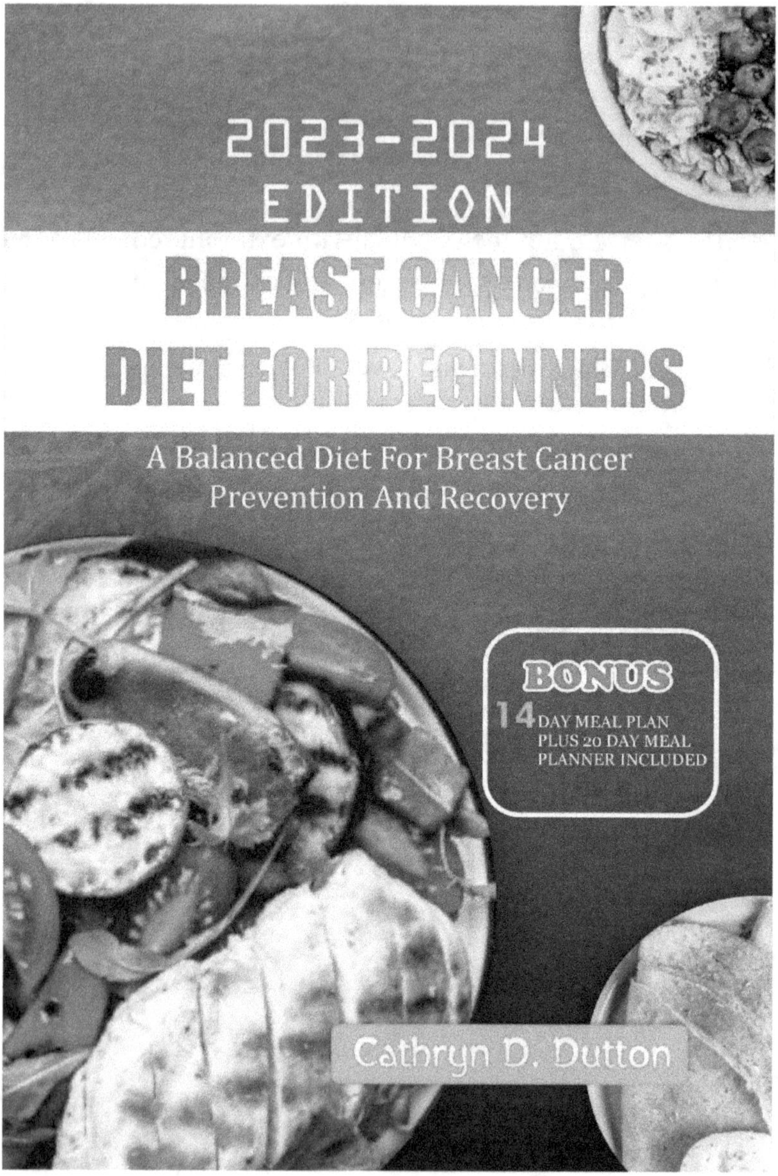

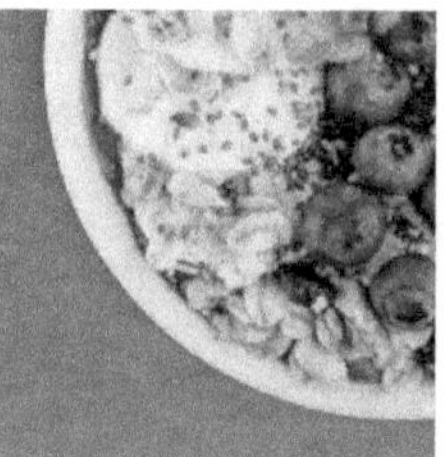

2023-2024
EDITION

BREAST CANCER
DIET FOR BEGINNERS

A Balanced Diet For Breast Cancer
Prevention And Recovery

BONUS
14 DAY MEAL PLAN
PLUS 20 DAY MEAL
PLANNER INCLUDED

Cathryn D. Dutton

1.Grilled Chicken with Roasted Vegetables

Ingredients

- 2 boneless, skinless chicken breasts
- Assorted vegetables (such as bell peppers, zucchini, carrots, and red onions), sliced Olive oil
- Salt and pepper
- Garlic powder
- Paprika
- Dried herbs (such as thyme, rosemary, or oregano)

Preparation

Preheat your grill to medium-high heat.

1. Season the chicken breasts with salt, pepper, garlic powder, and paprika on both sides.

2. Brush the chicken breasts with a bit of olive oil to prevent sticking and enhance flavor.

3. Place the seasoned chicken breasts on the grill. Cook for about 6-8 minutes on each side, or until the internal temperature reaches 165°F (75°C) and the chicken is no longer pink in the center.

4. The vegetables should be ready while the chicken is grilling. Sliced vegetables should be combined in a bowl with olive oil, salt, pepper, and any additional dried herbs you like.

5. Spread the seasoned vegetables on a baking sheet in a single layer.

6. Roast the vegetables in the oven at 400°F (200°C) for about 20-25 minutes, or until they are tender and slightly browned around the edges. You can also grill the vegetables in a grilling basket alongside the chicken.

7. When the chicken is cooked and the vegetables are broiled, eliminate them from the barbecue and broiler.

8. Serve the barbecued chicken with the broiled vegetables as an afterthought.

Go ahead and change the flavoring and selection of vegetables as indicated by your inclinations. Partake in your flavorful Barbecued Chicken with Simmered Vegetables!

2. Whole-Wheat Pasta Primavera

Ingredients

- Whole-wheat pasta, 8 ounces
- Olive oil, two teaspoons
- 2 minced garlic cloves
- 1 finely sliced tiny onion
- broccoli florets in a cup
- julienned 1 medium carrot
- finely sliced 1 medium red bell pepper
- sliced 1 medium zucchini
- 1 cup halved cherry tomatoes
- pepper and salt as desired
- Grated Parmesan cheese, 1/4 cup (optional)
- chopped fresh basil leaves as a garnish

Preparation

1. Follow the directions on the package to prepare the whole-wheat pasta. Drain, then set apart.

2. Olive oil should be heated in a large pan over medium heat. Add the minced garlic and cook until fragrant, about 1 minute.

3. When the onion is added, sauté it for two to three minutes, or until it begins to soften.

4. Fractured carrot and broccoli florets should be added to the skillet. Cook for a further 3 to 4 minutes while stirring occasionally.

5. Slices of red bell pepper and zucchini should be added to the skillet. Cook the veggies for a further 2 to 3 minutes, or until they are soft but still crisp.

6. The cherry tomato halves should be added and cooked for 1-2 minutes, or until they begin to soften.

7. Add salt and pepper to taste when preparing the vegetable combination.

8. Whole-wheat pasta that has been cooked should be added to the skillet and gently combined.

9. Grated Parmesan cheese can be added to the spaghetti and veggies, if preferred.

10. Hot Whole-Wheat Pasta Primavera should be served with fresh basil leaves cut on top.

11. Enjoy your Primavera Whole-Wheat Pasta, which is nutritious and colorful!

3. Stir-Fried Tofu and Broccoli

Ingredients

- 14 oz (400g) two cups of chopped, firm broccoli florets

- Vegetable oil, two teaspoons
- 2 minced garlic cloves
- 1 teaspoon finely chopped ginger
- 2/fourths cup soy sauce
- 1 tablespoon oyster sauce (for flavoring, if desired)
- 1 teaspoon cornstarch (to make the sauce thicker)
- 1/4 cup water or vegetable broth
- pepper and salt as desired
- (Optional) Red pepper flakes for heat
- Sesame seeds for decoration
- green onions, sliced, as a garnish

Preparation Method

1. Tofu should be prepared by draining it and wrapping it in a fresh kitchen towel. Put a weighted object on top to force out extra water. Unwrap the tofu and cut it into cubes after around 15 to 20 minutes have passed.

2. Making the sauce: Mix the cornstarch, soy sauce, oyster sauce (if using), and vegetable broth or water in a small bowl. Place aside.

3. Vegetable oil should be heated over medium-high heat in a large pan or wok.

4. Cubes of tofu should be added to the heated skillet. The tofu should be brown and somewhat crispy after cooking

for around 5-7 minutes while stirring occasionally. Tofu should be taken out of the pan and placed aside.

5. Stir-fry the vegetables: If extra oil is required, add it to the same pan. For about 30 seconds, add the minced garlic and ginger and sauté until fragrant. When the broccoli florets are brilliant green and just beginning to soften, add them and stir-fry for 3 to 4 minutes.

6. Return the cooked tofu to the skillet with the broccoli to combine with the veggies.

7. Pour the prepared sauce over the tofu and broccoli after giving it a short swirl. Toss everything to cover it all equally. A minute or two should pass as the sauce thickens.

8. Add seasoning and garnish: If you want the stir-fry to be spicy, add salt, pepper, and red pepper flakes. Combine by tossing.

9. To serve, place the stir-fried broccoli and tofu in a serving dish. Sesame seeds and thinly sliced green onions are garnishes.

Enjoy: Serve the stir-fried tofu and broccoli over cooked rice or noodles. Enjoy your delicious and nutritious meal!

4.Baked Salmon with Asparagus

- 4 fillets of salmon
- 1 clipped bunch of asparagus
- Olive oil, two teaspoons
- pepper and salt as desired
- 2 minced garlic cloves
- 1 sliced lemon
- fresh dill, if desired
- serving slices of lemon

Preparation

1. Turn on the oven to 400 °F (200 °C).
2. On a baking sheet that has been lightly oiled or lined with parchment paper, arrange the salmon fillets.

3. Place the salmon fillets and the trimmed asparagus on the baking sheet.
4. Sprinkle salt, pepper, and chopped garlic over the fish and asparagus after drizzling the olive oil over them.

5. Each salmon fillet should have a slice of lemon on top.
6. If preferred, top the salmon with fresh dill.

7. Bake for 12 to 15 minutes in the preheated oven, or until the salmon flakes easily when tested with a fork. The thickness

8. of the fillets may affect the cooking time.

9. When ready, take the food out of the oven and serve it hot with lemon wedges.

5. Chickpea and Vegetable Curry

Ingredients

- 1 can (15 oz) washed and drained chickpeas
- 1 finely chopped onion
- 2 minced garlic cloves
- 1 chopped bell pepper, 1 diced zucchini, 1 sliced carrot
- 1 cup chopped tomatoes, either fresh or canned
- coconut milk, 1 cup
- Curry powder, two teaspoons
- 1/9 cup cumin
- 1 teaspoon of cilantro
- Half a teaspoon of turmeric
- Cayenne pepper, 1/4 teaspoon (adjust to taste)
- Salt as desired
- 2 tablespoons oil (either vegetable or olive oil)
- garnish with fresh cilantro leaves
- Naan bread or cooked rice for serving

Preparation Method

1. Over medium heat, warm the oil in a big pan or pot.
2. The chopped onion should be added and sautéed until transparent.

3. Add the minced garlic and stir for a further one to two minutes, or until fragrant.

4. To the saucepan, add the chopped bell pepper, zucchini, and carrot. Cook the veggies for about 5-7 minutes, or until they begin to soften.

5. The veggies should be covered in a mixture of curry powder, cumin, coriander, turmeric, and cayenne pepper. The spices should be well mixed into the veggies.

6. Add the coconut milk and chopped tomatoes. To mix everything, stir.

7. Drain the chickpeas, then add them to the saucepan along with the veggies and coconut milk combination.

8. To taste, add salt to the dish. If you want the dish to be hotter or more flavorful, you may now change the spice proportions.

9. For around 15 to 20 minutes, simmer the curry over low heat with the lid on to let the flavors mingle and the veggies finish cooking.

10. Taste the curry when the flavors have formed and the veggies are soft, then check the seasoning and make any necessary adjustments.

11. Alternatively, serve the chickpea and vegetable curry with naan bread and boiled rice.
12. Before serving, garnish with fresh cilantro leaves.

6. Grilled Veggie and Goat Cheese Quesadillas

Ingredients

- 4 substantial flour tortillas
- 1 cup of goat cheese crumbles
- 1 sliced zucchini, 1 sliced red bell pepper, 1 sliced yellow bell pepper, 1 sliced thin red onion
- baby spinach leaves, 1 cup
- Olive oil, two teaspoons
- pepper and salt as desired
- chopped fresh herbs, such as basil, thyme, or oregano, are optional.

Preparation method

1. Preheat a grill or stovetop grill pan over medium heat.
2. Sliced zucchini, red, yellow, and red onions are combined with olive oil in a basin. Add salt and pepper to taste.

3. Grill the thinly sliced veggies for 4-5 minutes per side, or until they are soft and slightly browned. Take it off the grill, then place it aside.

4. On a spotless board, spread out the flour tortillas.

5. Goat cheese that has been shredded should be spread over one half of each tortilla.

6. Add some baby spinach leaves on top of the goat cheese.

7. Include the grilled veggies on top of the spinach.

8. Add some chopped fresh herbs to the veggies if you want for flavor, if preferred.

9. Over the contents, fold the tortillas in half to form a half-moon.

10. The tortillas should be golden brown and crispy and the cheese should be melted, then place the quesadillas on the grill or grill pan and cook for around 2-3 minutes on each side.

11. Before slicing, take the quesadillas from the grill and let them cool for a moment.

12. Serve heated quesadillas that have been cut into wedges.

13. Enjoy your mouthwatering Quesadillas with Grilled Veggies and Goat Cheese!

7. Cauliflower Rice Stir-Fry

Ingredients

- a single large head of cauliflower
- 2 tablespoons of oil (such as olive or vegetable oil)
- 1 cup of mixed veggies, such as carrots, peas, and bell peppers
- 2 minced garlic cloves
- 1 teaspoon finely chopped ginger
- 2/fourths cup soy sauce
- 1 optional tablespoon of oyster sauce
- pepper and salt as desired
- Sesame seeds and sliced green onions are optional garnishes.

Preparation Method

1. After cleaning, cut the stem and leaves from the cauliflower. Give it a floret cut.

2. The florets should be placed in a food processor and pulsed until rice-sized bits are formed. As an alternative, you may grind the florets into rice-like bits using a box grater.

3. In a large pan or wok, heat the oil over medium-high heat.

4. For about 30 seconds, add the minced garlic and ginger and sauté until fragrant.

5. The mixed veggies should be added and sautéed for a few minutes until they soften.

6. Add the cauliflower rice to the opposite side of the pan after pushing the veggies to one side.

7. For 3 to 4 minutes, stir-fry the cauliflower rice until it's soft but not mushy.

8. In the pan, mix the sautéed veggies and cauliflower rice.

9. To the pan, add the soy sauce and oyster sauce (if using). Combine everything and stir it thoroughly.

10. To taste, add salt and pepper to the food.

11. Allow the flavors to combine for a further 2-3 minutes of cooking.

12. Remove from heat and, if like, sprinkle with sesame seeds and finely chopped green onions.

13. Serve the delicious stir-fried cauliflower with rice as a main course or a side dish.

8. Baked Eggplant Parmesan

Ingredients

- 2 big eggplants, cut into rounds about 1/2 inch thick.
- Salt
- 2 cups of sauce marinara
- Shredded mozzarella cheese in two cups
- grated Parmesan cheese, half a cup
- all-purpose flour, half a cup
- Three big eggs
- 1 cup Italian-style breadcrumbs, ideally
- Olive oil is used to brush the slices of eggplant.
- sprigs of fresh basil, for decoration

Preheat your oven to 375°F (190°C).

1. Slices of eggplant should be salted on both sides and let to rest for about 30 minutes. By doing this, extra moisture and bitterness are eliminated. After 30 minutes, use paper towels to pat the eggplant slices dry.

2. Put together a breading station: Place the flour in a single, shallow dish. Beat the eggs in another bowl. Place the breadcrumbs in a third dish.

3. Each eggplant slice should be floured before being dipped into the beaten eggs and then breadcrumbs. Shake off extra material.

4. On baking pans, arrange the breaded eggplant pieces. Apply some olive oil on both sides. For 20 to 25 minutes, or until the eggplant is cooked through and golden brown, bake in the preheated oven. In the middle of baking, turn the slices over.

5. .

6. Spread a thin layer of marinara sauce in a baking dish.

7. Layer the prepared eggplant slices in the baking dish, slightly overlapping each layer to cover the bottom. More marinara sauce should be spooned over the eggplant pieces.

8. Over the sauce, strew a layer of grated Parmesan and mozzarella cheese.

9. With the remaining eggplant pieces, sauce, and cheeses, repeat the layering.

10. Bake in the oven for about 20 minutes with the baking dish covered with aluminum foil.

11. The cheese should be melted and bubbling after another 10-15 minutes of baking after removing the foil.

12. When ready, take it out of the oven and allow it cool before serving.

13. Before serving, garnish with fresh basil leaves.

9. Quinoa-Stuffed Bell Peppers

Ingredients

- 4 big, multicolored bell peppers
- 1 cup of rinsed and drained quinoa
- 2 cups of water or vegetable broth
- Olive oil, 1 tbsp
- 1 minced tiny onion
- 2 minced garlic cloves
- 1 cup chopped tomatoes, either fresh or canned
- 1 cup cooked black beans, either from a can or from dry beans.
- 1 teaspoon of cumin, ground
- 1 paprika teaspoon
- pepper and salt as desired

- 1 cup shredded cheese, your choice of cheddar or mozzarella
- chopped fresh cilantro or parsley as a garnish

Preheat your oven to 375°F (190°C).

1. Remove the bell peppers' tops, then scoop out the seeds and membranes. Place aside.

2. Bring the water or vegetable broth to a boil in a medium saucepan. For about 15 minutes, or until the quinoa is cooked and the liquid has been absorbed, add the quinoa, lower the heat to low, cover, and simmer. With a fork, fluff the quinoa and set it aside.

3. Olive oil should be heated in a large pan over medium heat. Add the chopped onion and simmer for three to four minutes, or until transparent. For one more minute, add the minced garlic.

4. Add the cooked black beans, chopped tomatoes, ground cumin, paprika, salt, and pepper. Allow the flavors to mingle for a further 3–4 minutes of cooking.

5. .

6. Mix everything together in the skillet after adding the cooked quinoa. If necessary, adjust the seasoning.

7. Put the quinoa mixture inside the bell peppers, carefully packing it within.

8. The filled bell peppers should be put on a baking dish. Slice a tiny chunk off the bottom of the shaky peppers to help them stand up straight.

9. Bake the baking dish in the preheated oven for about 25 to 30 minutes, or until the bell peppers are soft. Cover the baking dish with aluminum foil.

10. Each stuffed pepper should be placed back in the oven for an additional 5-7 minutes, or until the cheese is melted and bubbling, after removing the foil.

11. Before serving, take them out of the oven and allow them to cool somewhat.

Before serving, garnish with freshly cut cilantro or parsley.

10. Grilled Turkey Burgers with Sweet Potato Fries

Ingredients

- 1 pound of turkey, ground
- breadcrumbs, 1/4 cup
- 1/4 cup of onion, cut finely.
- 2 minced garlic cloves
- Oregano, dry, 1 teaspoon
- one tablespoon dried basil
- pepper and salt as desired
- Sandwich buns
- Slices of tomato, lettuce, and any additional toppings you like
- Sweet potato fries' ingredients are as follows:

- Peeled and sliced into fries, two big sweet potatoes
- Olive oil, two teaspoons
- 1 paprika teaspoon
- one-half teaspoon of garlic powder
- pepper and salt as desired

1. Ground turkey, breadcrumbs, minced garlic, minced onion, dried oregano, dried basil, salt, and pepper should all be combined in a bowl. Mix thoroughly.

2. Using a spatula, divide the mixture into patties and shape them to fit your hamburger buns. To keep the patties from ballooning up while cooking, make an indentation in the center of each one.

3. Heat your grill to a moderately hot setting. The turkey patties should be cooked through and have an internal temperature of 165°F (75°C) by placing them on the grill and cooking them for about 5 to 6 minutes on each side.

4. For the sweet potato fries, preheat your oven to 425°F (220°C) while the burgers are frying.

5. Sweet potato fries should be equally coated with olive oil,

6. paprika, garlic powder, salt, and pepper in a big bowl.

7. On a baking sheet covered with parchment paper, arrange the seasoned sweet potato fries in a single layer.

8. When the sweet potato fries are crisp and golden brown, bake them in the preheated oven for 20 to 25 minutes, rotating them halfway through.

9. Put your favourite toppings on the buns and assemble your turkey burgers.

10. Serve the sweet potato fries and grilled turkey burgers together.

To support general health, consider a variety of veggies, whole grains, lean meats, and healthy fats when choosing your supper. For individualized nutritional advice, speak with a healthcare practitioner.

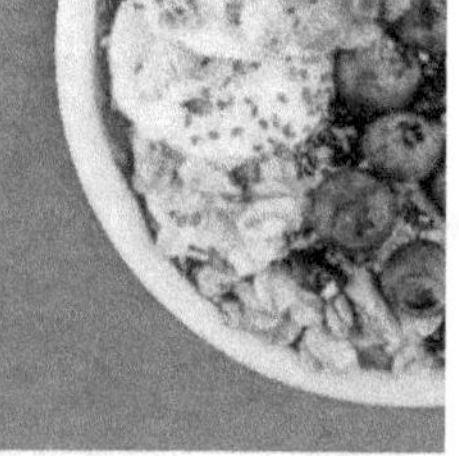

2023-2024
EDITION

BREAST CANCER
DIET FOR BEGINNERS

A Balanced Diet For Breast Cancer
Prevention And Recovery

BONUS
14 DAY MEAL PLAN
PLUS 20 DAY MEAL
PLANNER INCLUDED

Cathryn D. Dutton

1.Hummus and Veggie Sticks

Sure, here's a basic recipe for making Hummus and Veggie Sticks:

Ingredients for Hummus:

- 1 can (15 ounces) of rinsed and drained chickpeas
- Tahini (sesame paste), 1/4 cup
- Extra virgin olive oil, 1/4 cup
- 1-2 minced garlic cloves
- 1 or 2 lemons juice
- 1 teaspoon of cumin, ground
- Water, as needed and Salt, to taste

Ingredients for Veggie Sticks

- Banana sticks
- carrot sticks
- Cut cucumbers
- sliced bell peppers

Preparation:

Make Hummus:
a. Combine the chickpeas, tahini, olive oil, chopped garlic, lemon juice, cumin, and a dash of salt in a food processor.

b. If the mixture is too thick, gradually add water to get the right consistency.

c. Taste the dish and make any necessary seasoning adjustments by adding additional lemon juice, salt, or garlic.

Prepare Veggie Sticks:
a. Peel and wash the carrots. Prepare them as sticks..

b. After cleaning, slice the celery into sticks.

c.. Cucumber and bell pepper should be washed. They are cut into strips.

Serve
a. Put the vegetable sticks on a dish..
b. Center a dish of hummus there.
c.. For more flavor, you may add some paprika and pour some olive oil over the hummus.

Enjoy

Enjoy a nutritious and delectable snack by dipping the vegetable sticks into the hummus!

You are welcome to alter the recipe by incorporating your preferred herbs, spices, or more veggies into the hummus or by using other kinds of vegetables for the sticks.

2. Greek Yogurt and Berries

Ingredients

- Grecian yogurt
- Strawberries, blueberries, raspberries, blackberries, and other berries mixed together
- Optional honey for sweetness
- Optional granola or nuts for crunch

Preparation

1. The berries should be well washed and dried.

2. You may cut larger fruit like strawberries into bite-sized pieces if you'd like.

3. Add the required quantity of Greek yogurt to a bowl. You may change the amount to suit your tastes.

4. The yogurt should be topped with the mixed berries.

5. Drizzle some honey over the berries and yogurt for a hint of sweetness.

6. For added texture and taste, you may also want to sprinkle some chopped nuts or granola.

7. Depending on your preference, gently combine the ingredients or leave them stacked.

8. You may now eat your Greek Yogurt and Berries meal. It is delicious as a dessert, snack, or breakfast food.

9. You are welcome to change the quantities and ingredients to suit your preferences. Enjoy!

3. Trail Mix

Ingredients

- 1 cup of nuts, such as walnuts, almonds, cashews, or peanuts
- 1 cup of dried fruits, such raisins, cranberries, apricots, or cherries
- 1/2 cup of seeds, such as sunflower or pumpkin seeds
- 0.5 cups of optional chocolate chunks or chips
- Optional: 1/2 cup of oats, cereal, or pretzels
- a dash of salt, if desired

1. If preferred, roast the nuts and seeds in a dry pan over medium heat until they are aromatic and just beginning to turn brown. Be sure to let them cool before using.

2. Combine the nuts, seeds, dried fruit, chocolate chips (if using), and nuts in a mixing basin. Mix in any additional ingredients, such as oats, cereal, or pretzels.

3. To spread the ingredients equally, give the mixture a thorough toss.

4. If you prefer, season the mixture with a little salt to bring out the flavors.

5. For convenient snacking on-the-go, transfer the trail mix to an airtight container or individual snack-sized bags.

6. Feel free to alter the ingredients to suit your dietary restrictions and taste preferences. The handmade trail mix is delicious!

4. Apple Slices with Nut Butter

- 2 to 3 medium apples
- nut butter of your preference (such as cashew, peanut, or almond butter)

- Added extras include chopped nuts, raisins, honey, and cinnamon.

Preparation

1. The apples should be carefully cleaned and dried.

2. Apples should be cored and sliced thin. Peel them if you'd like, or leave the peel on for more fiber and nutrients.

3. Apple slices should be arranged on a serving platter.
4. Apply a small coating of the nut butter of your choice to each apple slice.

5. Pour honey over the nut butter if you'd like it to be sweeter.
6. For taste and texture, top with your preferred garnishes, such as chopped almonds, raisins, or a dash of cinnamon.

Enjoy your tasty and nourishing apple slices with nut butter right now!

To fit your tastes, feel free to be creative with the toppings and nut butter choices.

5. Whole Grain Crackers with Cheese

Ingredients

- Crackers made with whole grains (20–24 pieces).
- 1 cup shredded cheese, your choice of cheddar or mozzarella
- 1 teaspoon of thyme, rosemary, oregano dry herbs
- one-half teaspoon of garlic powder
- pepper and salt as desired

Preparation

Preheat your oven to 350°F (175°C).

1. Put the whole grain crackers on a baking sheet that has been prepared with silicone baking mat or parchment paper. Make sure they are separated equally and are not touching.

2. The grated cheese, dried herbs, garlic powder, salt, and pepper should all be combined in a bowl. Mix well to spread the ingredients evenly.

3. Each cracker should have a little quantity of the cheese mixture on it. Spread it out just enough to cover the cracker, leaving a thin border all the way around.

4. Bake the crackers and cheese on the baking sheet in the preheated oven. About 8 to 10 minutes of baking time should be used to melt and bubble the cheese.

5. The crackers should cool for a few seconds after the baking sheet is taken out of the oven. As it cools, the cheese will get firmer.

6. You may serve the crackers as a tasty snack or starter once they have somewhat cooled.

6. Kale Chips

Ingredients

- brand-new kale leaves
- Almond oil
- (Optional) Salt
- spices of your choosing (such as chili flakes, nutritional yeast, and garlic powder)

Preparation

Preheat your oven to 300°F (150°C).

1. The kale leaves should be well cleaned and dried. You may use paper towels or a salad spinner.

2. Each kale leaf should have its rough stem removed before being torn into bite-sized pieces.

3. Sprinkle some olive oil over the kale leaves in a mixing dish.

4. To get an equal covering, lightly toss the leaves. Avoid using too much oil since it may cause the chips to get mushy.

5. Optionally, season the kale leaves with a bit of salt and your preferred spices. Garlic powder, nutritional yeast, or chili flakes are typical spices.

6. On a baking sheet, arrange the oiled kale leaves in a single layer. Depending on how much kale you use, more than one baking sheet can be required.

7. The kale chips should bake for 10 to 15 minutes in a preheated oven, or until crisp and gently brown. Keep an eye on them since they are prone to burning.

8. When the kale chips are finished, take the baking sheet out of the oven and allow them cool slightly before serving.

Enjoy your homemade kale chips as a healthy and flavorful snack!

7. Popcorn with Herbs

Ingredients

- popcorn kernels, 1/2 cup
- two tablespoons of butter or oil
- 1 teaspoon dry herbs, preferably a combination of rosemary, thyme, and oregano.
- Salt as desired

Preparation Method

1. Over medium heat, melt the butter or olive oil in a big saucepan. Allow butter to fully melt if using.

2. Make sure the popcorn kernels are uniformly placed in a single layer before adding them to the saucepan. Put a cover on the saucepan.

3. The kernels will begin to pop as they warm up. To promote even popping and prevent scorching, give the pot a little shake every so often.

4. Remove the saucepan from the heat when the popping stops. For one minute, keep the lid on to let any last kernels burst.

5. Sprinkle the dry herbs over the heated popcorn while it's still hot. The herbs will adhere to the popcorn better thanks to the remaining heat.

6. To equally distribute the herbs, gently shake the pot or toss the popcorn with a spatula.

7. To make sure the spice is well spread, season to taste with salt and toss one more.

8. Before savoring your tasty popcorn with herbs, let it cool a little.

9. Keep in mind that you may vary the amount of salt and herbs to suit your taste. Enjoy your tasty pleasure of handmade popcorn!

8. Chia Seed Pudding

Ingredients

- Chia seeds, 1/4 cup
- 1 cup milk, either dairy or plant-based (such as soy, coconut, or almond)
- Depending on how sweet you want it, use honey, maple syrup, or agave.
- Optional: fresh fruits, cinnamon, vanilla flavor, and nuts as garnish

Preparation

1. Chia seeds and milk should be mixed in a bowl. Make sure the chia seeds are spread equally by thoroughly combining.

2. Add your preferred sweetener and any other flavors, such as cinnamon or vanilla extract. To blend, fully stir.

3. Place the bowl in the refrigerator for at least two to three hours and ideally all night. The chia seeds will absorb the liquid during this time and take on a pudding-like consistency.

4. Give the pudding a thorough stir once it has had time to set in order to remove any possible clumps.

5. Chia seed pudding should be served in small dishes or glasses. Fresh fruit and nuts can be sprinkled on top to give it more taste and texture.

6. Take pleasure in your filling chia seed pudding.
7. Feel free to alter the recipe to your liking by using your preferred fruits, nuts, or other garnishes.

9. Edamame

Ingredients

- Edamame pods, either frozen or fresh
- (To taste) salt

Preparation Method

1. Bring water in a big saucepan to a boil. Sprinkle a little salt into the water.
2. When the water is boiling, add the edamame pods and cook them for three to five minutes, or until they are soft.

Follow the cooking time recommendations on the package if using frozen edamame.

3. When the edamame pods are finished cooking, strain them and place them right away in a dish of cold water. Their brilliant green color is preserved and the cooking process is stopped.

4. When the edamame pods have cooled, rinse them once more and use a paper towel to pat them dry.

5. Add salt to taste to the cooked edamame pods and toss to coat well.

6. As a snack or starter, put the edamame pods in a dish and serve. Simply remove the edamame beans from their pods and place them in your mouth to devour.

Enjoy your tasty and healthy edamame!

Note: You can also experiment with different seasonings or dips for added flavor.

10. Cottage Cheese with Pineapple

Ingredients

- 1 cup of cubed cottage cheese
- 1 cup of pieces of fresh pineapple
- 1 tablespoon butter or olive oil
- one tablespoon of ginger paste
- one tablespoon of garlic paste
- 1/4 cup cumin seeds
- One-half teaspoon of turmeric powder
- Red chili powder, 1/2 tsp. (modify to taste)
- Salt as desired
- 1 tablespoon of finely chopped cilantro (coriander leaves)

Preparation Method

1. In a pan, melt the butter or olive oil over medium heat.
2. The cumin seeds should be added and let a little moment to crackle.

3. Ginger and garlic paste should be added. Sauté until fragrant for one minute.

4. Red chili powder and turmeric powder should be added. Mix thoroughly.

5. For two to three minutes, add the fresh pineapple chunks and heat them until they start to soften.

6. As you mix the spices and pineapple together, add the cubed cottage cheese (paneer).

7. Cook the cottage cheese for a further 2 to 3 minutes while stirring periodically.

8. Add salt to taste and combine thoroughly.

9. Add chopped cilantro (coriander leaves) as a garnish.

10. Serve the hot cottage cheese and pineapple as a side dish with rice or toast after removing from the heat.

Enjoy your Cottage Cheese with Pineapple!

Note: You can adjust the spice levels and sweetness by varying the amount of red chili powder and pineapple used.

These snack suggestions emphasize nutrient-dense foods that help support a diet that is both balanced and healthful. Always pay attention to your body's signals of hunger and pick foods that suit your particular nutritional requirements.

2023-2024
EDITION
BREAST CANCER
DIET FOR BEGINNERS
A Balanced Diet For Breast Cancer
Prevention And Recovery
BONUS
14 DAY MEAL PLAN
PLUS 20 DAY MEAL
PLANNER INCLUDED
Cathryn D. Dutton

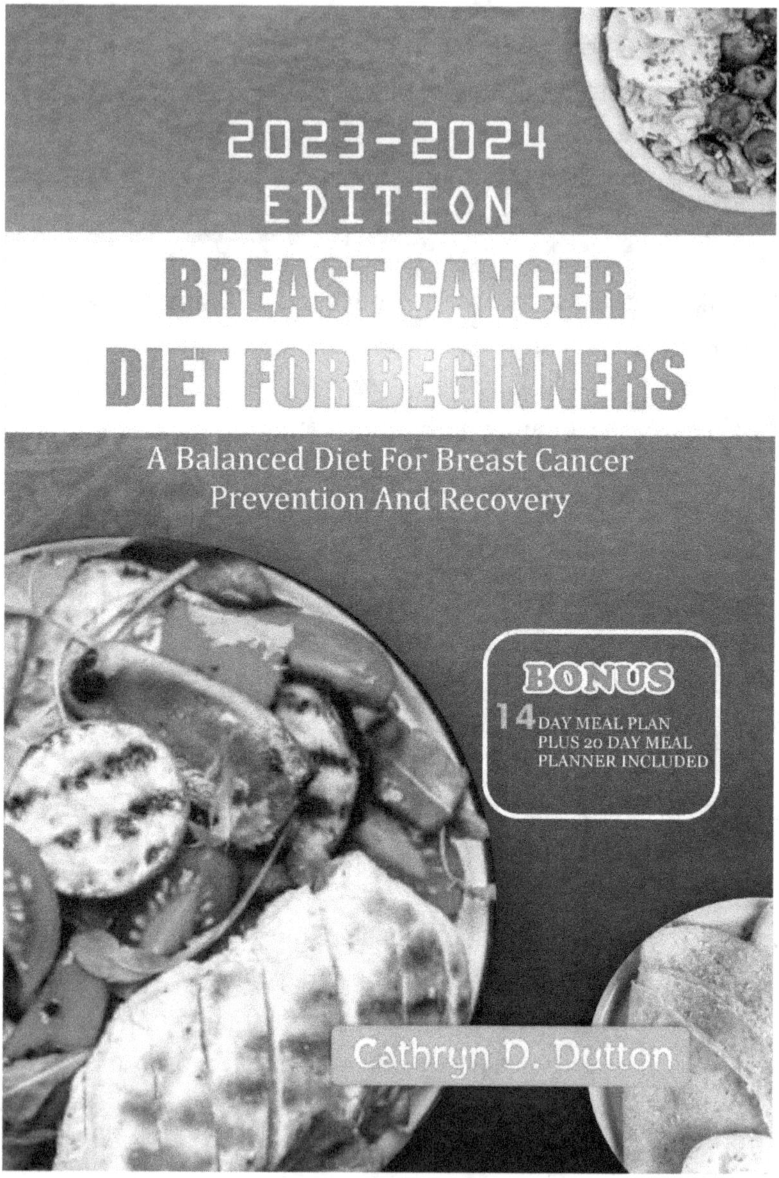

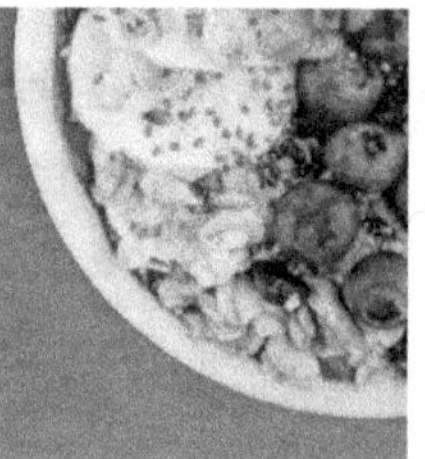

1.Mixed Berry Parfait

Ingredients

- Strawberries, blueberries, raspberries, and other berries totaling 1 cup
- 2 cups of Greek yogurt (or another type of yogurt)
- 14 cup of granola
- two teaspoons of maple syrup or honey (optional)
- Fresh mint leaves can be used as a garnish.

Preparation Method

1. The berries were washed and dried. If using strawberries, slice them after removing the stems.

2. Yogurt and honey or maple syrup (if used) should be thoroughly mixed in a bowl.

3. Start stacking the parfait in bowls or serving glasses. Place a tablespoon of the yogurt mixture in the bottom to start.

4. To the yogurt, add a layer of mixed berries.

5. Granola should be scattered on top of the fruit.

6. Once the glasses or bowls are full, stack the ingredients once again, finishing with a yogurt layer.

7. As a garnish, add some more berries and mint leaves to the parfaits.

8. Before serving, place the parfaits in the refrigerator for at least 30 minutes to let the flavors to mingle.

9. Take pleasure in your mouthwatering Mixed Berry Parfait for breakfast or dessert!

10. Any other ingredients, such as chopped nuts, seeds, or even a drizzle of chocolate sauce, are welcome to be added to the recipe to suit your tastes.

2. Dark Chocolate-Dipped Strawberries

Ingredients

- dried and rinsed fresh strawberries, chopped dark chocolate (at least 70% cacao),
- White chocolate may be used to drizzle.
- Optional garnishes include chopped nuts, sprinkles, or shredded coconut.

1. Use parchment paper to cover a baking sheet.
2. In a bowl suitable for the microwave, slowly melt the dark chocolate for 20 to 30 second intervals, stirring in between, until smooth. Alternately, use a stovetop double boiler.

3. Swirl the melted chocolate over a strawberry while holding it by the stem, coating roughly two thirds of it. Let the extra chocolate trickle off.

4. On the prepared baking sheet, put the strawberry that has been dipped. With the remainder of the strawberries, repeat the procedure.

5. If using, melt some white chocolate and use it to decorate the strawberry dip.

6. You may cover the strawberries with chopped almonds, sprinkles, or crushed coconut while the chocolate is still soft.
7. For faster results, put the baking sheet in the refrigerator or let the chocolate set at room temperature.

8. The strawberries should be gently removed from the parchment paper once the chocolate has completely hardened and arranged on a serving platter.

9. The strawberries covered in dark chocolate can be served right away or kept for a few hours in a refrigerator.

Enjoy your luscious strawberries coated in dark chocolate.

3. Baked Apples with Cinnamon

Ingredients

- 4 medium-sized apples, such as Honeycrisp or Granny Smith
- quarter cup brown sugar
- 1 teaspoon of cinnamon powder
- 2 teaspoons softened butter
- optional 1/4 cup chopped nuts, such as walnuts or pecans
- 1/4 cup optional dried cranberries or raisins
- For serving, vanilla ice cream or whipped cream is optional.

Preparation

Preheat your oven to 350°F (175°C).

1. The apples should be carefully cleaned and dried. Remove the apples' cores and seeds with an apple corer or a tiny knife to leave a hollow hole in the middle.

2. Brown sugar, cinnamon powder, melted butter, chopped nuts, and raisins or dried cranberries, if used, should all be combined in a small bowl.

3. Fill the empty spaces of each apple with the cinnamon mixture by gently pushing it down.

4. The filled apples should be put on a baking dish. You may add a little additional cinnamon on top if you'd like.

5. Bake the dish in the preheated oven for about 25 to 30 minutes, or until the apples are soft, with the foil covering. Depending on the size and type of apples you use, the baking time may change.

6. After baking, take the apples out of the oven and let them cool somewhat before serving.

7. Warm baked apples can be served either by themselves or, if preferred, with a scoop of vanilla ice cream or a dollop of whipped cream.

8. Take pleasure in your mouthwatering Baked Apples with Cinnamon!

4. Frozen Banana Pops

Sure, here's a simple recipe for Frozen Banana Pops:

Ingredients

- Bananas that are ripe (1–2)
- Popsicle sticks or skewers made of wood
- Dark, milk, or white chocolate chips or melted chocolate
- toppings of your choosing, such as crushed coconut, sprinkles, or chopped almonds.

Preparation Method

1. Bananas should be peeled and split in half crosswise. To make a banana pop, insert a wooden skewer or popsicle stick into either side of the fruit.

2. The banana pops should be frozen for at least one to two hours, or until they are solid, on a plate or tray coated with parchment paper.

3. The chocolate should be heated in a double boiler or in a microwave-safe bowl while the banana pops are frozen. Stir the chocolate regularly until it is completely melted and smooth.

4. After the banana pops have frozen, dip them one by one into the melted chocolate, coating them evenly with a spoon. Let the extra chocolate trickle off.

5. If desired, roll the chocolate-covered banana pops in your preferred toppings, such as crushed coconut, chopped almonds, or sprinkles.

6. Return the chocolate-covered banana pops to the plate or tray that has been lined with paper, and freeze them for a further 30 minutes to let the chocolate to solidify.

7. Your frozen banana pops are prepared when the chocolate has completely hardened. Any leftovers should be frozen in an airtight container.

5. Chia Seed Pudding with Fruit

Ingredients

- Chia seeds, 1/4 cup
- milk, either dairy or non-dairy, such as almond, coconut, etc., 1 cup
- 1 tablespoon sweetener (such as agave nectar, honey, or maple syrup).
- One-half teaspoon of vanilla extract
- Fresh fruit (such as berries, banana slices, mango, etc.)
- optional nuts or seeds for topping

Preparation

1. Chia seeds, milk, sugar, and vanilla essence should all be combined in a bowl. To properly combine the ingredients, stir them well.
2. To avoid clumping, give the mixture another toss after letting it settle for about 5 minutes.

3. For at least two hours or overnight, cover the bowl and place in the refrigerator. Chia seeds will begin to soak up the liquid during this time, giving the mixture a pudding-like consistency.

4. Make sure the chia pudding is thoroughly blended by giving it a quick swirl just before serving.

5. Pour the chia pudding into dishes or glasses for serving.
6. Add fresh fruit of your choice and nuts or seeds on top for some extra crunch.

7. Take pleasure in your tasty and nourishing Chia Seed Pudding with Fruit!

8. You are welcome to make the recipe your own by adding your preferred fruits, nuts, and sweeteners.

6. Fruit Salad with Mint

Ingredients

- a variety of fresh fruits, including oranges, grapes, kiwis, pineapple, watermelon, and strawberries.
- brand-new mint leaves
- (Optional) Honey or maple syrup for sweetness
- (Optional) Lime or lemon juice for tanginess

Preparation Method

1. As necessary, wash and peel the fruits. Remove the cores, seeds, and pits. Fruits should be chopped into bite-size pieces.

2. Finely chop the fresh mint leaves.
3. Combine the diced fruits and mint leaves in a large mixing dish.

4. Pour honey or maple syrup, if desired, over the fruit mixture to give it more sweetness.

5. To intensify the tastes, squeeze lime or lemon juice over the fruit.

6. Toss the fruits and mint leaves together gently to combine and evenly distribute the honey, syrup, and citrus juice.
7. Refrigerate the fruit salad for at least 30 minutes to enable the flavors to mingle. Cover the bowl with plastic wrap or a lid.

8. Give the fruit salad one last toss just before serving to properly distribute the juices and flavors.
9. Fruit salad should be served in separate bowls or cups.

Enjoy your mint-infused, cool fruit salad!

7. Yogurt and Berry Parfait

Ingredients

- Greek yogurt, either vanilla or plain
- a variety of berries, including strawberries, blueberries, and raspberries
- Honey for granola (optional)
- Mint leaves, used as a garnish

Preparation

1. As required, wash and cut the berries.

2. Start by adding a tablespoon of Greek yogurt to the bottom of serving glasses or bowls.

3. To the yogurt, add a layer of mixed berries.

4. Granola should be scattered on top of the fruit.

5. When you reach the top of the glass, continue layering until you reach a layer of berries.

6. Pour some honey over the top layer if you'd like it to be sweeter.

7. Add a mint leaf as a garnish for a cool touch.

Enjoy your tasty yogurt and berry parfait right away!

Depending on your preferences and the size of the serving containers, feel free to change the amounts of each component. Enjoy your delicious and nutritious parfait!

8. Frozen Grapes

Sure, here's a simple recipe for frozen grapes

Ingredients

- Grapes (any variety)
- Water

Preparation

1. The grapes should first be properly washed in cold running water. With a paper towel or kitchen towel, pat them dry.

2. If the stems are still there, cut the grapes off them.

3. On a parchment-lined baking sheet, spread the grapes out. Make sure they are arranged in a single layer and are not touching.

4. The grape-filled baking sheet should be put in the freezer. Allow them to freeze for a minimum of two to three hours, or until they are fully solid.

5. The frozen grapes can then be placed in an airtight container or a plastic bag that can be resealed.

6. Prior to eating them, keep the frozen grapes in the freezer.
7. On a hot day, frozen grapes are a delightful and cooling snack!

9. Oatmeal Banana Cookies

Ingredients

- 2 mashed ripe bananas
- rolled oats, 1 cup
- One-half teaspoon of vanilla extract
- 1/8 teaspoon cinnamon powder
- 1/4 cup optional chocolate chips or raisins
- 14 cup optionally chopped nuts, such as walnuts or almonds

Preparation

1. Preheat your oven to 350°F (175°C) and line a baking sheet with parchment paper.

2. The mashed bananas, vanilla essence, and ground cinnamon should all be combined in a mixing dish. Combine well after mixing.

3. The rolled oats should be well mixed with the banana mixture before being added.

4. Add the raisins, chocolate chips, and chopped nuts, if desired. Mix the ingredients until the dough is equally spread.

5. Drop spoonfuls of the dough onto the prepared baking sheet, a few inches apart, using a spoon or your hands.

6. With the back of the spoon or your fingertips, softly press down on each biscuit.

7. Bake in the preheated oven for 12 to 15 minutes, or until the edges of the cookies are golden brown.

8. When the cookies are done, take the baking sheet out of the oven and let them cool on the sheet for a short while before

9. moving them to a wire rack to finish cooling.

10. savor your wonderful oatmeal banana cookies!

10. Homemade Fruit Sorbet

Ingredients

- 2 cups of fruit, such as berries, mangos, peaches, etc., either fresh or frozen
- Granulated sugar, 1/2 cup (modify to taste)
- a half-cup of water
- 1 tablespoon of optionally added lemon juice for taste and tartness

Preparation

Make a basic syrup first by combining sugar and water in a pot. Stirring constantly, heat over medium heat until the sugar is fully dissolved. Remove from heat once dissolved, then allow to cool to room temperature.

a. Get the fruit ready

The fruit you're using should be cleaned, peeled, and checked for seeds or pits. If necessary, chop the fruit into tiny pieces.

b. Blend the fruit:

In a blender, combine the diced fruit, cooled simple syrup, and any more lemon juice. Blend until a purée is smooth.

c. Optional

Strain the fruit puree through a fine mesh strainer to get a smoother texture by removing any lumps or seeds. This step is not required.

Refrigerate the fruit combination for at least an hour, or until it is cold, to cool the mixture.

d. Churn the sorbet

If you have an ice cream machine, churn the ingredients in accordance with the manufacturer's directions until it resembles sorbet. You may create ice cream by hand using the instructions below if you don't have an ice cream maker.

e. Manual Churning Method:

Fill a small container with the cold fruit mixture.

The container should be put in the freezer.

Use a fork to aggressively whisk the liquid once every 30 minutes to smash any ice crystals that develop.

Continue doing this for another two to three hours, or until the sorbet is creamy and smooth.

e. Final freeze:

Transfer the sorbet to an airtight container and freeze it for a few hours or until it is hard, depending on your preference for firmness.

Serving: Before serving, let the sorbet to soften a little by allowing it to sit at room temperature. Enjoy by scooping into bowls or cones.

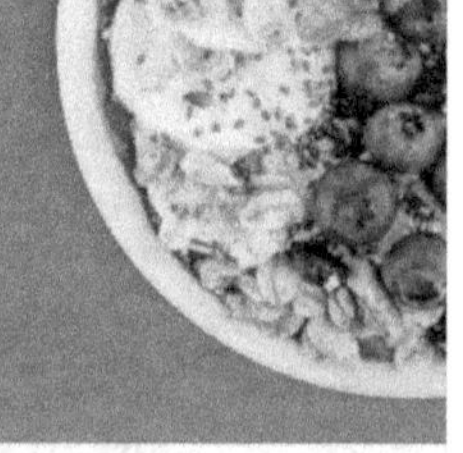

2023-2024
EDITION
BREAST CANCER
DIET FOR BEGINNERS
A Balanced Diet For Breast Cancer
Prevention And Recovery
BONUS
14 DAY MEAL PLAN
PLUS 20 DAY MEAL
PLANNER INCLUDED
Cathryn D. Dutton

Here's a 14-day meal plan using the options you've provided

Day 1
Breakfast: Berry Smoothie Bowl
Lunch: Grilled Vegetable Salad
Dinner: Grilled Chicken with Roasted Vegetables

Day 2
Breakfast: Oatmeal with Flaxseeds
Lunch: Mediterranean Chickpea Bowl
Dinner: Whole-Wheat Pasta Primavera

Day 3
Breakfast: Avocado Toast
Lunch: Broccoli and Almond Stir-Fry
Dinner: Stir-Fried Tofu and Broccoli

Day 4
Breakfast: Greek Yogurt Parfait
Lunch: Lentil and Spinach Soup
Dinner: Baked Salmon with Asparagus

Day 5

Breakfast: Chia Seed Pudding
Lunch: Salmon and Quinoa Bowl
Dinner: Chickpea and Vegetable Curry

Day 6

Breakfast: Spinach and Mushroom Egg Scramble
Lunch: Kale and Walnut Salad
Dinner: Grilled Veggie and Goat Cheese Quesadillas

Day 7

Breakfast: Salmon Breakfast Wrap
Lunch: Tuna and White Bean Salad
Dinner: Cauliflower Rice Stir-Fry

Day 8

Breakfast: Turmeric Scrambled Tofu
Lunch: Veggie Wrap with Hummus
Dinner: Baked Eggplant Parmesan

Day 9

Breakfast: Whole-Grain Pancakes
Lunch: Brown Rice Sushi Rolls
Dinner: Quinoa-Stuffed Bell Peppers

Day 10
Breakfast: Fruit Salad with Nuts
Lunch: Black Bean and Sweet Potato Burrito
Dinner: Grilled Turkey Burgers with Sweet Potato Fries

Day 11-14: You can repeat the meal plan from Days 1-4 for Days 11-14 or mix and match to create variations based on your preferences.

Remember to adjust portion sizes and ingredients based on your dietary needs and goals. Additionally, ensure you're drinking plenty of water throughout the day and consider incorporating healthy snacks between meals if needed.

CONCLUSION

In conclusion, a healthy, balanced diet can be extremely important for managing and preventing breast cancer. You may provide your body the nutrition it needs to maintain general health and perhaps lower your risk of breast cancer by including a range of colorful fruits and vegetables, lean meats, whole grains, and healthy fats in your regular meals. Additionally, keeping a healthy body weight, abstaining from excessive alcohol use, and limiting your intake of processed foods can all help to promote the health of your breasts. The importance of a healthy diet should never be overlooked, but it should always be a part of a larger lifestyle that includes periodic screenings, stress reduction, and exercise on a regular basis. You may empower yourself in the battle against breast cancer and advance your general wellbeing by adopting a proactive attitude to your health.

Sincere thanks from the bottom of our hearts for choosing to read the "Breast Cancer Diet Cookbook for Beginners." We applaud your dedication to good health and are honored to participate in your gastronomic exploration.

You've taken positive action toward living a better, happier life by reading these pages. Your commitment to taking care of your body and promoting breast health is impressive and motivating.

Remember that each meal you cook is a show of self-care and a testimonial to your fortitude and resiliency as you set out on this culinary adventure. One delicious meal at a time, we're rewriting the story of breast health together.

We appreciate your participation in this crucial mission. Here's to your health, one delicious meal at a time.

With heartfelt thanks,
[CATHRYN DUTTON] and the Cookbook Team

Cathryndutton03@Gmail.com

14 DAY
MEAL PLANNER

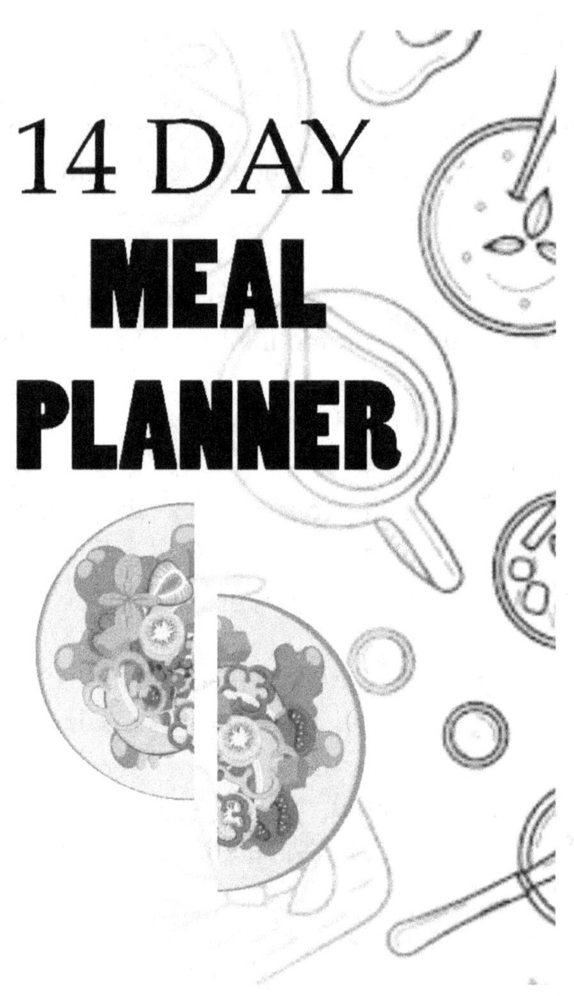

Menu List:

Breakfast

Lunch

Dinner

Important Meal;

shopping list:

To Do List

....
....
....
....
....

- ....
- ....
- ....
- ....
- ....

Notes And Tips

Menu List:

Breakfast

Lunch

Dinner

Important Meal:

shopping list:

To Do List

Notes And Tips

Menu List:

Breakfast

Lunch

Dinner

Important Meal:

shopping list:

To Do List

Notes And Tips

Menu List:

Breakfast

Lunch

Dinner

Important Meal;

shopping list:

To Do List

● ....

● ....

● ....

● ....

● ....

To Buy

salad

Notes And Tips

Menu List:

Breakfast

Lunch

Dinner

Important Meal:

shopping list:

To Do List

Notes And Tips

Menu List:

Breakfast

Lunch

Dinner

Important Meal:

shopping list:

To Do List

Notes And Tips

Menu List:

Breakfast

Lunch

Dinner

Important Meal;

shopping list:

To Do List

....

....

....

....

....

Notes And Tips

Menu List:

Breakfast

Lunch

Dinner

Important Meal;

shopping list:

To Do List

Notes And Tips

Menu List:

Breakfast

Lunch

Dinner

Important Meal:

shopping list:

To Do List

Notes And Tips

Menu List:

Breakfast

Lunch

Dinner

Important Meal;

shopping list:

To Do List

Notes And Tips

Menu List:

Breakfast

Lunch

Dinner

Important Meal;

shopping list:

To Do List

Notes And Tips

Menu List:

Breakfast

Lunch

Dinner

Important Meal:

shopping list:

To Do List

....
....
....
....
....

- ....
- ....
- ....
- ....
- ....

Notes And Tips

Menu List:

Breakfast

Lunch

Dinner

Important Meal;

shopping list:

To Do List

....
....
....
....
....

Notes And Tips

Menu List:

Breakfast

Lunch

Dinner

Important Meal:

shopping list:

To Do List

Notes And Tips

Menu List:

Breakfast

Lunch

Dinner

Important Meal:

shopping list:

To Do List

Notes And Tips

Menu List:

Breakfast

Lunch

Dinner

Important Meal;

shopping list:

To Do List

Notes And Tips

salad

TO BUY

Menu List:

Breakfast

Lunch

Dinner

Important Meal;

shopping list:

To Do List

Notes And Tips

Menu List:

Breakfast

Lunch

Dinner

Important Meal:

shopping list:

-
-
-
-
-

To Do List

Notes And Tips

www.ingramcontent.com/pod-product-compliance
Lightning Source LLC
Chambersburg PA
CBHW070809260726
48660CB00005B/1784